D0648173

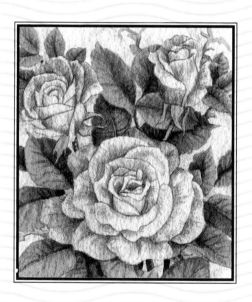

THE AURA OF LOVE

INSPIRING ROSE

PUBLICATIONS INTERNATIONAL, LTD.

Louis Weber, C.E.O.
Publications International, Ltd.
7373 North Cicero Avenue
Lincolnwood, Illinois 60646

Permissions never granted for commercial purposes.

Manufactured in China.

8 7 6 5 4 3 2 1

ISBN: 0-7853-3413-0

Dawn Baumann Brunke has a degree in massage therapy from the Potomac Institute of Myotherapy and practices aromatherapy. She is editor of *Alaska Wellness* magazine and has authored many articles on holistic healing. Ms. Brunke wrote the introduction and profile text of this publication.

Cara Filipeli is an accomplished poet. She has contributed to a poetry anthology entitled *Inspirations*. Her work appears on pages 33 and 58.

Margaret Anne Huffman is an award-winning writer and journalist. She has authored and co-authored inspirational titles including *Second Wind* and *Simple Wisdom*. She has also contributed to *Graces*, *Family Celebrations*, and *365 Daily Meditations for Women*. Ms. Huffman's work appears on pages 25, 26, 34, 41, 45, and 53.

Laurel Kallenbach is a freelance writer and poet. She has a master of arts degree in creative writing from Syracuse University and is former senior editor of *Delicious!* magazine. Ms. Kallenbach's work appears on pages 38 and 48.

Other material compiled by:
Helen H. Moore, Kelly Boyer Sagert, and Kelly Womer

Note: This book does not constitute the practice of medicine. If you have any health questions or concerns, the publisher suggests you consult your doctor.

Aromatherapy:

An Introduction

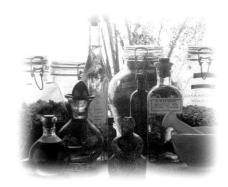

How easy it is to become lost in the intoxicating fragrance of a flower garden, the pungent awakening of spices and dried herbs, the crisp burst of scent from a freshly peeled orange, or the sweet intensity of a newly bloomed rose. Aroma has the power to inspire, sedate, energize, and entice.

Aroma is also a link to other times and places. The sharp, earthy smell of burning leaves recalls dis-

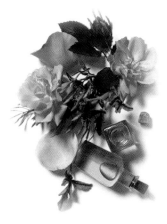

tant autumns; the aroma
of gingerbread cookies
conjures childhood mem-
ories; and the lingering
perfume of a lover's scent
summons the warm clasp
of a close embrace.

Aroma means scent, but it has powers beyond
those that arouse or arrest the senses. Within the
fragrances of aromatic plants are substances that
improve health, promote healing, and support your
general well-being. These substances are found in the
plant's essential oils, which are responsible for its
unique fragrance as well as its healing benefits.

But aromatherapy doesn't work by the sense of
smell alone. Essential oils can be used topically, taking

direct action on surrounding tissues and entering the bloodstream to be carried throughout the body.

The modern world has newly discovered the enchanting magic of aroma as well as the potent healing gifts contained in essential oils. These gifts, though, have been used by mankind at least since biblical times, and probably before. Today we understand why and how essential oils treat psychological and physical illness. In ancient times, people just knew that they worked.

THE ANCIENT MEANING AND USE OF SCENT

Mysterious, invisible, and deeply moving, aroma was long believed to hold the soul of a plant, to be the essence of the divine. The Egyptians believed the

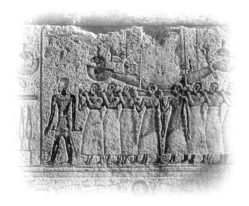

fleeting scent of a plant was a metaphor for the human soul. Ancient peoples believed deities would find prayers more pleasing when sweetly scented, and so the musky wisps of incense were used in nearly every culture to carry prayers heavenward. The ancients surrounded themselves with the richness of aroma, believing that as scented air entered their lungs and pores, a link was forged to the divine. In ancient Greece, oracles inhaled incense scented with bay leaves to inspire their visions, and Tibetan women captured aromatic clouds of cedar smoke to propel them into prophecy. Purifiers of body and soul, fragrant billows of smoke were also used to induce tranquility, insight, intoxication, and inner peace.

Ancient peoples also learned that heated animal fats could absorb the aromatic properties of fragrant flowers and leaves. When cooled, such concoctions were found to help heal wounds, soothe sore muscles, protect skin from the elements, and add a scent of mystery and allure to the wearer. It was later discovered that fragrance could be held in water as well, either to be ingested as a tonic or applied as scent to the skin and hair.

The Egyptians were famous for their scented oils. So masterfully did they blend essential oils that calcite pots once filled with their scented creations still held a faint aroma when the tomb of King Tutankhamen was opened 3,000 years later. The Romans bathed in fragrance, while the Greeks generously applied scented oils to their bodies. The East Indians turned the use of scent into a sensual art form. Women anointed their glistening, freshly bathed bodies with jasmine, sweet patchouli, amber, musk, sandalwood, and saffron. Each part of the body held a different scent, an aromatic garden of earthly delights.

The bewitching aspects of aroma are as old as the entanglement of love and power. Cleopatra lured Mark Anthony as her slaves burned incense and fanned the smoke into the sails of her ship. When the Queen of Sheba made her famous visit to King Solomon, it was to discuss the trading of fragrant resins. Delicately scented smoke was used to perfume

a woman's hair
in ancient Japan,
and geishas
measured their
customer's stay
by the number
of incense sticks
that were burned.

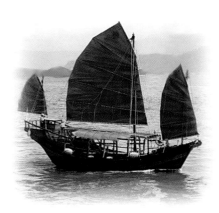

Ancient Athens was famous for merchants selling enticingly scented body oils, musks, aromatic perfumes, and disks of fragrant incense. The Phoenicians traded exotic wares of Chinese camphor, Indian cinnamon, and sandalwood. Aromatics merchants from India and Persia carried jasmine-scented sesame oil to China, while rosewater was mixed into the mortar used to build sacred mosques in the East. So was the world once connected by the pervasive and persuasive power of fragrance.

Aromatherapy Today

Today, aromatherapy has come of age. Offering not only sensual pleasure but a fragrant cure, essential oils are once again being used for their health benefits.

Enter, then, the provocative world of aroma with its incredible diversity of scent, from the seductive richness of jasmine to the sweet gentleness of lavender, from the tangy scent of citrus to the floral purity of rose. Whether you choose a scent to invigorate and exhilarate or refresh and soothe, aromatherapy is an exquisite journey into body, mind, and soul.

ROSE

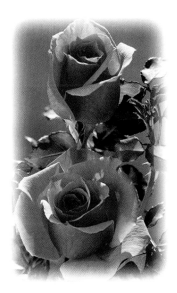

With its tall, thorny stem and lavish layers of soft, velvety blossoms, the rose has been considered the queen of flowers since ancient times. It has long been symbolic of love and beauty because of its exquisite form and alluring scent. Traditionally, the red rose symbolizes passion and the white rose purity. Romance and innocence: These are rose's twin motifs.

There are many legends about the exalted rose, but it is most often linked with the Greek goddess of

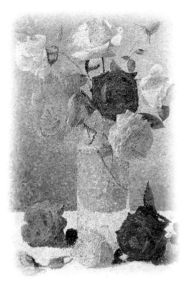

love and beauty, Aphrodite. Some myths contend that the flower originally sprang from Aphrodite's tears, while others say the rose was a gift from the gods as she emerged from the foamy sea at birth. Later, as Aphrodite pursued her lover, she pricked her finger on a thorny rosebush and her blood colored the flowers a deep red. Rearrange the letters that spell Eros, the name of Aphrodite's son, and you will also find the rose.

The lovely rose can grow wild and carefree, blooming in rambling overgrown hedges, or it can be painstakingly pruned. Remarkably hardy, roses grow in many types of soils all over the world. In fact, there are more than 250 different species and more than 10,000 hybrids. Three varieties, however, are most often used for their enchanting aroma: the French rose, or *Rosa gallica;* the cabbage rose, or *Rosa centifolia;* and the damask rose, or *Rosa damascena.*

It was in ancient Persia and Rome that the rose was first cultivated. The elegant flower with the heavenly fragrance was later brought by Turkish merchants to Bulgaria, where the best and most expensive rose oil is now produced. Rose blossoms contain only a very small amount of essential oil, and it takes 30 roses to make a single drop of Bulgarian rose oil. An extravagant 60,000 roses are needed to make a mere ounce of the distilled essence, and 10,000 pounds of rose blossoms are necessary to produce just one pound of oil!

Regardless of price, there is tremendous demand for the rose's lavishly sweet, floral scent. Newly bloomed flowers are hand-picked in the cool, early morning hours, and a two-phase distillation process yields a small quantity of essential oil and a larger amount of rose water, which is a by-product of distillation.

Sweet and gentle, the rose was used by Cleopatra in a variety of beauty rituals. And, when Cleopatra met Mark Antony, rose petals were strewn eight inches deep on the ground. The ancient Greeks and Romans macerated fresh roses in hot fat to produce scented pomades. In Egypt, pomades were similarly made, but fashioned into large cones and worn on the top of the head. Body heat would melt the fat, thus unleashing the fragrance to mingle with the hair and the skin on the face and neck.

Legend credits the discovery of rose oil to the wedding feast of Persian princess Nour-Djihan. The tale says that, as she was being rowed through a canal strewn with rose petals during the wedding procession, Nour-Djihan swept her hand through the water. The warmth of the sun had caused the oil from the petals to float on the water's surface, and when the princess withdrew her hand from the water, it was covered in sweetly scented perfume. Thus alchemists in the kingdom learned the secret of

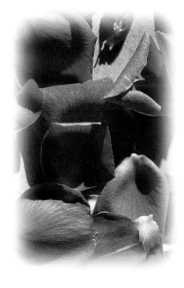

extracting the precious essential oil of roses.

The healing tradition of the rose is in many ways linked to its mythic association with love, purity, and romance. Its slightly spicy, arousing scent stimulates all the senses and, like the emotion of love itself, can bring an initial rush of intoxication. However, rose also calms the emotions and soothes the soul. Rose oil strengthens the heart, emotionally and spiritually. It instills compassion, heals emotional wounds, and comforts those in despair. Rose encourages us to love again, even if trust has been broken.

Extract of rose has been used traditionally for headaches and tired eyes. Rose oil has also been used widely as a primary ingredient in creams and lotions, not only for its scent but also for its mild antiviral properties. Oil of rose is especially suitable for treating dry, inflamed, and sensitive skin. As rose water is mildly astringent, it is also helpful for cleaning, toning, and refreshing sensitive skin. Rose is known to be a cell rejuvenator, suitable for all types of complexions. It is among the most antiseptic of all essential oils.

The shape of the rose and its distinctly feminine bouquet seem to imply its efficacy in treating female problems. Indeed, rose-scented massage oil works wonders for a variety of feminine conditions, from cramps to the moodiness of premenstrual syndrome and menopause. Rose is also used to alleviate anxiety, tension, irritability, and depression.

The naturally evocative scent of rose exudes the joy of possibility. The depth of its fragrance speaks to a richness of physical beauty and also of spirit and soul. The rose has an aura of mysterious sweetness.

The rose's robust floral fragrance is timeless. With deep, healing qualities and a profoundly rich, sweet scent, the rose will continue to inspire love, ardor, elegance, and confidence.

ANTI-AGING COMPLEXION CREAM

15 drops geranium oil
3 drops rose oil
2 drops frankincense or neroli oil
2 ounces complexion cream

Stir the essential oils into the cream. Use daily.

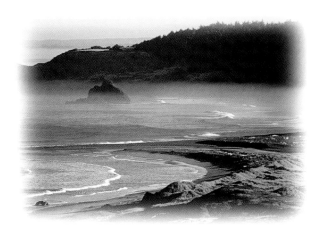

There are two births; the one when light

First strikes the new awakened sense;

The other when two souls unite,

And we must count our life from thence:

When you loved me and I loved you

Then both of us were born anew.

—WILLIAM CARTWRIGHT

It is difficult to define love. But we may say that in the soul, it is a ruling passion; in the mind, it is a close sympathy and affinity; in the body, a wholly secret and delicate longing to possess what we love— and this after much mystery.

—François, Duc de la Rochefoucauld

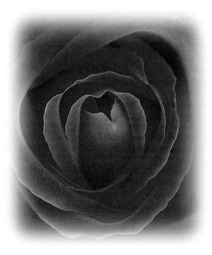

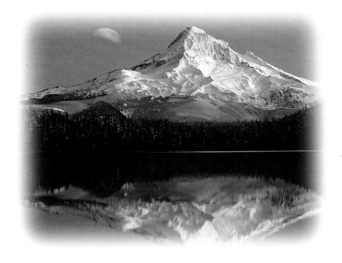

Love has the power of snowflakes that fall softly and gently yet become a glacier.

Like a wedding band, love encircles but doesn't bind.

Solid like rock, it is a bridge, not a wall.

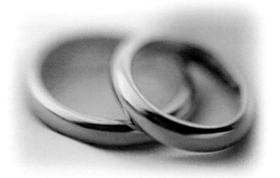

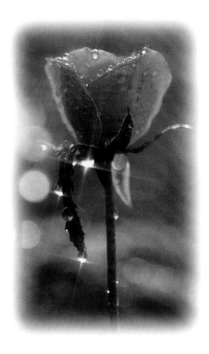

One word frees us of all the weight and pain in life.

That word is love.

—SOPHOCLES

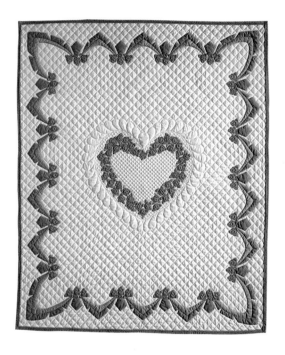

Love is a cloth which imagination embroiders.

—Voltaire

"What else

Is love, but the most noble, pure affection

Of what is truly beautiful and fair,

Desire of union with the thing beloved?"

"I have read somewhere, that man and woman

Were, in the first creation, both one piece,

And being cleft asunder, ever since

Love was an appetite to be rejoined."

—BEN JONSON

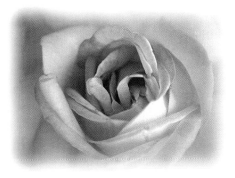

love is more thicker than forget

more thinner than recall

more seldom than a wave is wet

more frequent than to fail

it is most mad and moonly

and less it shall unbe

than all the sea which only

is deeper than the sea

love is less always than to win

less never than alive

less bigger than the least begin

less littler than forgive

it is most sane and sunly

and more it cannot die

than all the sky which only

is higher than the sky

—E.E. CUMMINGS

Flowers may beckon towards us,

but they speak toward heaven and God.

—Henry Ward Beecher

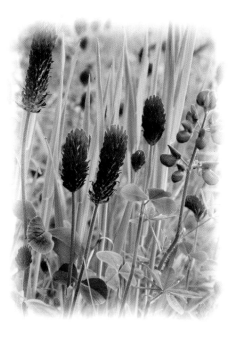

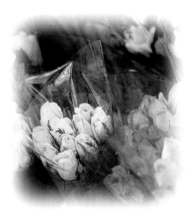

Once I wondered where love was,

I waited for it,

I wrote about it,

I talked about it,

I dreamed of it.

Then I found the recipe:

For every one part received,

you give two parts back.

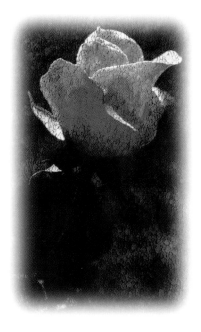

Affection, like fine vintage furniture, develops a rich

patina from years of faithful use.

Though we travel the world over to find the beautiful, we must carry it with us or we find it not.

—RALPH WALDO EMERSON

Let

Fate do her worst; there are relics of joy,

Bright dreams of the past, which she

cannot destroy;

Which come in the night-time of sorrow and care,

And bring back the features that joy used to wear.

Long; long be my heart with such

memories fill'd!

Like the vase, in which roses have

been distill'd—

You may break, you may shatter the vase

if you will,

But the scent of the roses will hang 'round

it still.

—Thomas Moore

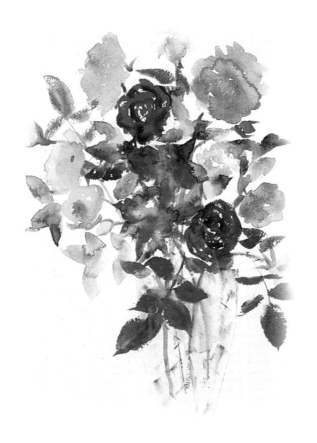

What hidden wonders the world offers:

an apple blossom newly opened

on the slender branch,

the way the butterfly brushes a stamen,

the impossibly soft landing of a snowflake

on the windowsill.

These are reminders that the universe

can only be loved inch by inch;

It's the minute that makes it glorious.

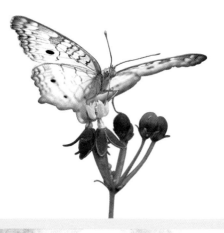

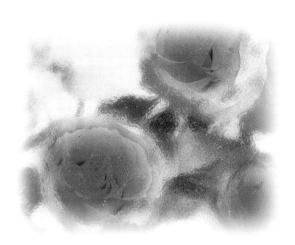

It is only with the heart that one can see rightly;

what is essential is invisible to the eye.

—Antoine de Saint-Exupéry

There are no little events with the heart.

It magnifies everything; it places in

the same scales the fall of an empire

of fourteen years and the dropping

of a woman's glove, and almost always

the glove weighs more than the empire.

—Honoré de Balzac

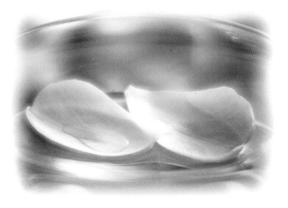

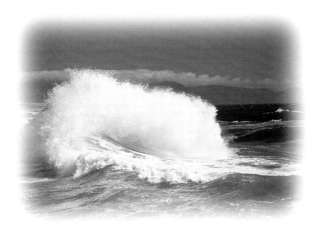

Age-blessed companions, they smile across the

years of practice, no words needed.

No one can understand the ebb and flow of life

as well as one who rides the same wave

at just a slightly different spot and is committed

to sharing the view.

Every word of every tongue is

Love telling a story to her own ears. . .

Love courses through everything,

No, Love *is* everything

How can you say, *there is no love,*

when nothing but Love exists?

All that you see has appeared because of Love.

All shines from Love,

All pulses with Love,

All flows from Love—

No, once again, all *is* Love

—FAKHRUDDIN 'IRAQI

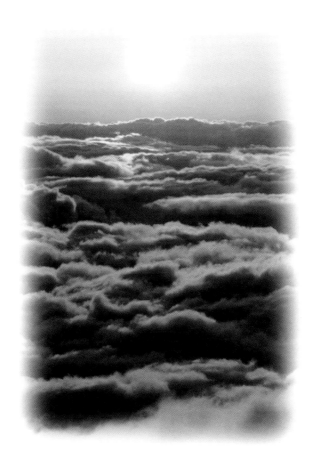

At the touch of love, everyone becomes a poet.

—PLATO

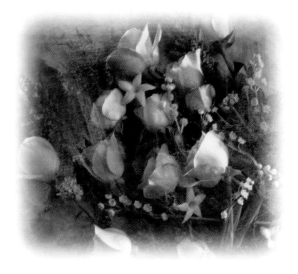

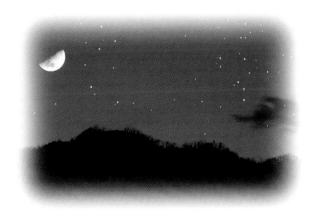

Firefly flashes on the night sky,

like individual gestures of love,

appear small when viewed one by one.

But collectively they reveal a darkness transformed.

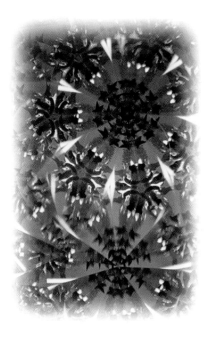

Love doesn't just sit there, like a stone,

it has to be made, like bread;

re-made all the time, made new.

—Ursula K. LeGuin

In a full heart there is room for everything, and in an empty heart there is room for nothing.

—ANTONIO PORCHIA

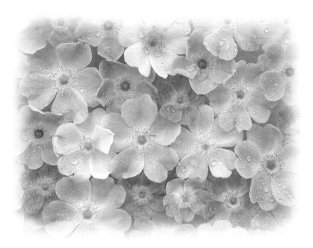

A lifetime of windswept sand has

sculpted the lovers

until their flesh is one.

For years his spine curve slept in the small

of her back. They're two

pieces of earth, puzzle-locked

into the eternal geology of love.

They've weathered together and are layered

with the twilight colors of ancient sediment.

They sigh in tandem breaths

like frail whispers of air through the canyon.

When shadows stretch, the two will fade

into the rust of day.

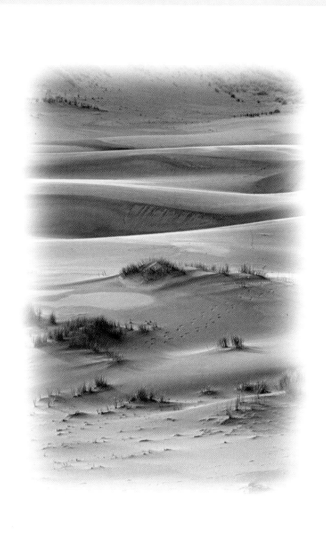

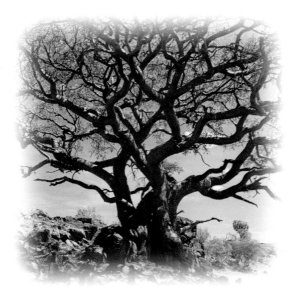

ove should be a tree whose roots are deep in the

earth, but whose branches extend into heaven.

—BERTRAND RUSSELL

Memory is the power to gather roses in winter.

—Anonymous

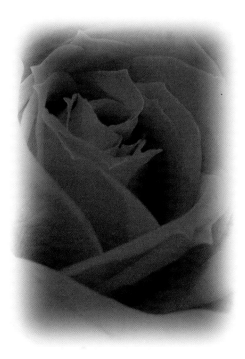

It would take a whole book to consider love,

for there is the very personal love for a dog or a cat,

and the love of life that surges suddenly

when you see the first evidence of spring in

the delicate snowdrops bending ivory blossoms

above the lacy snow.

—GLADYS TABER

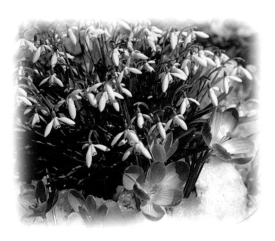

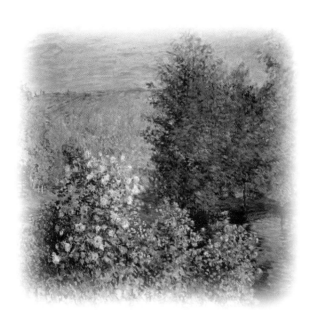

Love held onto remains seed; love shared becomes

both flower and fruit.

love is a place

& through this place of

love move

(with brightness of peace)

all places

yes is a world

& in this world of

yes live

(skillfully curled)

all worlds.

—E.E. CUMMINGS

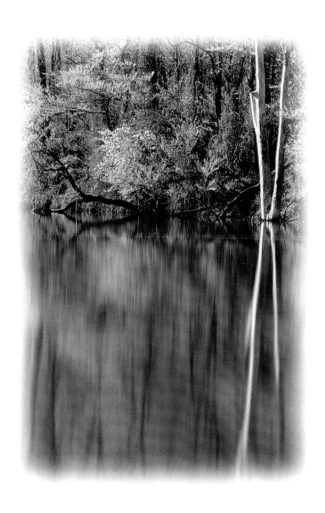

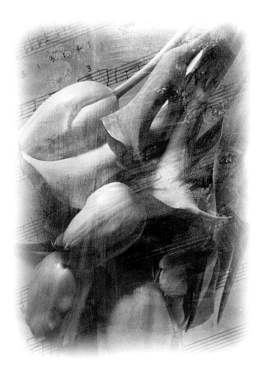

Whatever makes an impression on the heart seems

lovely in the eye.

—Sa'di

Love does not consist in gazing at each other,

but in looking together in the same direction.

—ANTOINE DE SAINT-EXUPÉRY

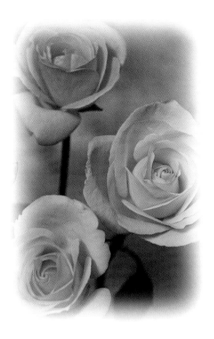

Love is like a rose. Each year when it blooms,

the color is just a shade different.

You have to notice the difference in each bloom

to take joy in the next.

Who would give a law to lovers?

Love is unto itself a higher law.

—BOETHIUS

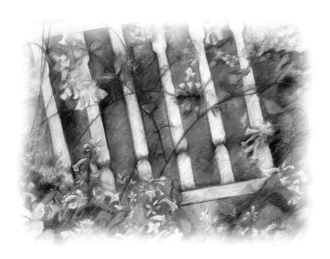

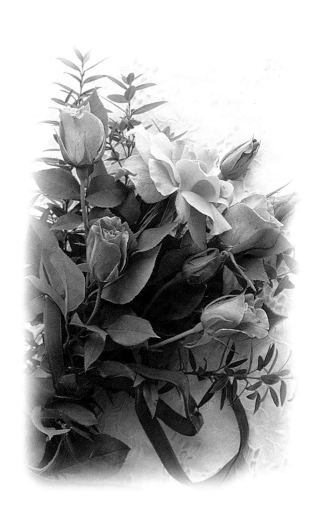